# Contents

Throughout this book you will notice little symbols next to some of the hints.  The symbols mean:

 Treats

 Things to make you feel better

 Things to help your relationship

 Information you need to know

 Things to think about

 Things you must do

This book is dedicated to the women that supported me, and to those that support you now.

BTL

ocf/10

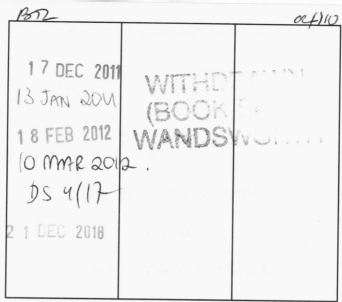

17 DEC 2011

13 JAN 2011

18 FEB 2012

10 MAR 2012 .

DS 4/17

2 1 DEC 2018

This book should be returned/renewed by
the latest date shown above. Overdue items
incur charges which prevent self-service
renewals. Please contact the library.

**Wandsworth Libraries**
**24 hour Renewal Hotline**
**01159 293388**
**www.wandsworth.gov.uk**  Wandsworth

L.749A (2.07)

| LONDON BOROUGH OF WANDSWORTH | |
|---|---|
| 9030 00000 9434 8 | |
| Askews | 29-Apr-2010 |
| 618.1453 PARK | £7.00 |
| | WWX0006283/0252 |

Cover image © Roger Otto I Agency: Dreamstime.com

Published by:
The Hysterectomy Association
Prospect House
Peverell Avenue East
Poundbury
Dorchester
Dorset, DT1 3WE

ISBN 10: 09532445 3 9
ISBN 13: 978-0-9532445-5-3

# Introduction

My own hysterectomy took place when I was thirty two; it changed my life. Before it, I was constantly ill, had serious problems with both endometriosis and IBS (irritable bowel syndrome) and would spend days every month in extreme pain. After it, I was suddenly well and I have never looked back, even though I couldn't have children.

But, I didn't know then, what I know now. I didn't know about the weight gain, the possible side effects of HRT, how tired I would be after the operation, when I could go back to work, what exercise I should (and shouldn't) do, and how much I would suffer from water retention. There were so many things I needed to know, but didn't and there were so many things I could have done to make my recovery easier, but didn't. What has always surprised me though is that even today, twelve years on; I'm still being asked these same questions by the thousands of women that contact The Hysterectomy Association every year. 101 Handy Hints for a Happy Hysterectomy was written to answer this need and hopefully it will provide you with some answers to the most common and frequently asked questions; as well as giving you some hints on how to make your recovery a successful one.

These hints are not designed to give you all of the information that is available; they are designed simply to raise your awareness so that you can then find out more about those things that matter. They are not in any particular order, although they are loosely divided into five sections: preparing for hysterectomy, getting ready to go into hospital, now you're in hospital, recovery at home and long term health. I would recommend reading through the whole book once and highlighting those that you might like to go back to later on. I would like to say thank you to everyone that has had a part in creating this book and mostly to the women that have contributed to the knowledge it contains, through their hints and tips for making every hysterectomy a happy one.

The Hysterectomy Association began life as a thesis for a Masters degree in Information Science. The women that took part in the research all asked for a source of information and support that was just for them. It has been running since 1987, mostly on a voluntary basis, and I hope that you will find the information in this book, and the others we have produced, useful in helping you to make some major decisions about your own future health.

Although much of this book represents current medical opinion, some of the information and resources listed in this book are by definition, outside the scope of generally accepted medical standards of care. They may be non-conventional, alternative or complementary. The information and resources listed should not be used in any way to provide a diagnosis or to prescribe any medical treatment. As in the case of conventional medicine, indiscriminate use of some therapies presented, without medical supervision may be harmful to your health. Individuals reading this material should in all cases, consult their own doctor or health practitioner for the diagnosis and treatment of medical conditions. The author and publisher will not accept responsibility for illness arising out of failure to seek medical advice from a doctor.

# Preparing for Hysterectomy

## 1. Be Prepared

Tom Lehrer, a mathematician from Harvard in the 1950's, wrote a somewhat degenerate song called Be Prepared[1].

*If you're looking for adventure of a new and different kind*
*And you come across a girl scout, who is similarly inclined*
*Don't be nervous, don't be flustered, don't be scared*
*Be prepared!*

Although the Boy Scout in question obviously had other, more risqué adventures in mind we can still learn from him.  As you read through this book, you will be pointed to 'girl scouts' who are 'similarly inclined' and by sharing your knowledge and concerns, you will find you are definitely less nervous, flustered and scared.

## 2. Becoming Informed ⓘ✓

This is one time in your life when information counts and getting enough of it will depend on how much you already know.  As we often say at The Hysterectomy Association, "you don't know what you don't know" and because of that simple fact asking questions becomes difficult as health professionals can assume that you already know everything because you aren't asking questions - and so the loop goes round and round.  You've taken the first positive step by purchasing this book.  These hints and tips will give you some ideas, but everyone is different and you will want answers to questions that are particularly relevant to your own set of circumstances, so you may find that some hints are more relevant than others.

Find some more good books, search the internet and ask other women what their experiences were. But be aware, not all information is 'good' information and some can be positively 'bad'. As you read and listen, note down more questions to ask your doctor, and when you do get an answer don't forget to write it down.

## 3. Find your support network ✍✓

We all need help some of the time but one thing many of us aren't good at, is asking for help when we are having a hysterectomy, and yet this is one of the most important ways we can help our recovery.

Your support network is going to be made of lots of people and might include your immediate family and friends; people you can call on, or pay, to do household chores and the school run; supermarket delivery services and maybe even the social services if you live alone and don't feel able to manage.

Everyone's support network is going to be different as we all have different needs and priorities, so thinking about what sort of help you might need and for how long is vitally important. One good way of deciding on your needs is to make a list of the various things you do in a 'normal' week. These might include shopping, ironing, looking after children and working. Some of them you will be able to disregard for the time being, like work, because you'll be taking time off to recover, but others will be on-going whatever your state of health. You may also find that you need to plan in advance for special occasions, such as Christmas and birthdays. Once you have your list, you can then think about how best to manage the activities and then you can set up the right system to support you.

## 4. To fill or not fill the freezer, that really is the question! ✍

One woman told me that when she had her hysterectomy the surgeon brought his patients into hospital on Sunday night and surgery was scheduled for the following Tuesday. He did this so that they could have a rest because they were always so tired from trying to get home and family organised.

Unfortunately the NHS doesn't allow us the luxury of a couple of days of bed rest before surgery these days, and I suspect that many of us still feel we have to make sure everyone copes while we're away. However, I have yet to talk to anyone that says their family went hungry because they hadn't filled the freezer before they had their hysterectomy.

There may be some virtue though, in organising yourself for when you get home from hospital, particularly if you live alone. A couple of weeks worth of healthy frozen meals and delivery of an organic farm box full of fruit and vegetables, when you get home, should make even the most health conscious of us feel virtuous. You may have already picked up, or had sent to you, the menus from all the takeaways that deliver in your area, or even found someone in the 'phone book that makes, and delivers, healthy nutritious meals. Even better would be training your partner and family not to assume you're going to disappear into a 'phone box, twirl round three times and emerge in a Superwoman outfit the very day you return from hospital!

## 5. Getting fit or fitter ☺✍

This isn't really about losing weight; this is about making sure your body is in the best possible condition to undergo surgery. At the same time you might also find that getting fitter improves some, or all, of your symptoms.

What about improving your lung and heart capacity through some sort of aerobic exercise, just enough to increase your normal heart rate for a few minutes every day. No, I'm not suggesting a Jane Fonda Workout, but why not put on some funky music and have a dance around the sitting room each day.

Giving up, or cutting down, on your cigarettes if you are smoker has to be a 'no brainer' really. Improving your diet, increasing your intake of water and walking a little every day will ensure your joints and muscles are in tip-top condition.

Exercise can also help to manage any pain you may have; it does this through the release of endorphins, the bodies natural painkillers. Other ways to release endorphins include laughter, deep relaxation and reducing stress levels; all good ideas when you are about to have surgery don't you think?

## 6. Diet, Schmiet! ☺✍

'You are what you eat' and if you eat junk food, your body won't be in the best condition to help you recover after your hysterectomy; if you do have a little weight to lose, then before your operation is the time to do it if you can. Not only will you recover more quickly afterwards, but you will minimise the strain on your heart and other vital organs while you are anaesthetised.

An easy way to get the best out of your body and your diet is to try and stick to the 'five a day' rule, eating at least five different portions of fruit and vegetables a day. It can be easy to incorporate them if you also link them to colours; red tomatoes, green peppers, oranges, purple sprouting broccoli ... the list is endless (almost). If cooking all this seems like a chore, then why not use a juicer or blender, add your five chosen pieces of fruit or vegetables at one go and drink your way to health; simple and effective.

## 7. Exploring complementary medicine ⓘ

In many ways a hysterectomy can provide you with the motivation to take stock of your life and look at how you might have contributed to your current state of health. Can you change the prognosis through your diet? Do you really need to have this surgery? You might be surprised at the number of medical conditions that seem to have poor diet as a contributory factor.

As well as diet, there are a number of complimentary therapies that may also have a positive impact on your health. Acupuncture for instance is a well known method of pain management; reflexology and aromatherapy techniques can promote relaxation and could therefore help those conditions made worse by stress. Simply drinking more water can help to flush toxins out of the body, and combining it with one of natures anti-inflammatories and antiseptics such as Aloe Vera[2], which is reputed to heal both internal and external wounds, can be hugely beneficial.

## 8. Coping with Fear ✍

At times like this it could be easy to be overcome by your fears; fears that often aren't talked about, or even admitted to, in many cases. But, it is surprising how much better you feel when you do confront the fears you have about your hysterectomy because it helps you put them into perspective.

So what are your fears? Writing them down and admitting the worst that you think can happen, can help you to prepare yourself physically, emotionally and mentally.

Try this exercise one day when you have an hour or two to yourself. Gather together paper and pens and put them on a side table; then sit in your favourite chair and close your eyes. Imagine yourself in a beautiful garden, see the plants and flowers, smell the scents, touch the petals and slowly feel your body relaxing. When you are fully relaxed open your eyes and think about the worst things that could happen as a result of your operation; write them down as they come into your mind and try not to analyse them before getting them down on paper.

Once you have written down as much as you can think of, close your eyes again, imagine the garden and slowly relax your body. When you feel relaxed, open your eyes and read through the list you have written down. Now think about what you can do to find out more about each of the things you have identified. This may involve talking to your GP, family and friends, it may involve a bit of research on the internet or at your local library. As you find out more information write it down, you will find that you feel more in control and the fears, although they may still be there, will become manageable and you will also find that you are less stressed, and a calmer person finds it easier to recover from a hysterectomy.

> Fear is often a fear of the unknown so banish the unknown with knowledge.

## 9. Join a support group ☺

There are many advantages to joining a support group of some description, including the fact that hysterectomy is not one of the most popular subjects over coffee at work! Sometimes it can be difficult to identify other women that have had one as they often don't want to talk about it - this is a shame as you can learn so much from other women's experiences.

However, despite these problems, there are many ways to get the support of your fellow women. One of the best ways of getting support is by using one of the internet discussion groups to ask the daftest questions and get encouraging, informative answers from other women who are just a few weeks or months ahead of you and who may have a different way of managing your problem. Most of these groups are free to join, have fantastic archives full of interesting conversations and you can just 'lurk' for a few days, weeks or months to see what is going on before plucking up courage and joining in. They also have the benefit that it may be a quicker way to get an answer to a problem than waiting to see your GP. Why not try our forums at *http://www.hysterectomy-association.org.uk/forums/*.

## 10. Ten questions to ask your gynaecologist ⓘ ✍

1. Have I had all the necessary diagnostic tests?
2. Why are you recommending a hysterectomy?
3. Are there any alternative forms of treatment open to me?
4. What organs will you be removing and why?
5. Will I have abdominal (horizontal or vertical) or vaginal surgery?
6. How long do you expect me to be in hospital?
7. Will I need to take HRT and what are the pros and cons?
8. What type of anaesthetic can I have?
9. What are the long term consequences of having a hysterectomy?
10. What are the risks associated with a hysterectomy?

## 11. Alternative treatments ⓘ ✍

You may have heard about the many alternative treatments that are now available for some conditions and it is worth talking to your GP and gynaecologist about whether any of them are suitable for you. Their availability will depend on a number of factors including whether there is anyone trained to perform them in your area, whether they are appropriate for your particular set of health problems and whether they have been licensed for use in the UK by NICE (National Institute for Clinical Excellence).

The reasons you might consider an alternative treatment (if it is available) will be different for everyone, but they might include whether you have completed your family or not, whether you are prepared to try complementary medicine or if you are concerned about the possible increased risk of heart disease or osteoporosis if your ovaries are removed.

### 12. Do I need my ovaries and cervix removed? ⓘ ✎

Removal of the ovaries [3, 4] and cervix [5, 6] has been a standard part of the hysterectomy operation in the UK for many years, however there is an increasing body of evidence that suggests that their removal is not necessary if they are healthy and not involved in your medical condition.

Removal of the ovaries will cause you to experience an immediate menopause, if you haven't already gone through it. Removal of the cervix *may* have an impact on how intensely you experience orgasm after your hysterectomy, although most women say that this isn't an issue. For many conditions, such as fibroids, heavy bleeding and prolapse there may be no medical reason to remove either the ovaries or the cervix and you should discuss your options with your gynaecologist.

The reason often given for their removal is that it helps prevent a possible problem in the future, but unless you're at high risk of developing cervical or ovarian cancer then you may feel this isn't a good enough reason to remove them while they are still healthy, and of course, keeping your ovaries will mean that you won't have to consider the pros and cons of HRT immediately. If you do keep your cervix, then you will continue to need regular cervical smears.

## 13. Start your question list ⓘ ✎ ✓

Obviously all the reading you are doing is going to be helping because this will identify issues that you hadn't thought about before, but will you remember to ask the questions when you actually see your GP or gynaecologist?

Buy a small notebook and keep it, and a pen, with you at all times. When you think of a question, write it down. Then, when you see your doctor you can nonchalantly flip open your notebook and stun him with your competence and knowledge. Not only that but you can write the answers down to refer back to later.

If you're feeling a bit nervous about asking your Doctor all these questions then take a friend or your partner along to appointments with you and they can make sure you ask the questions and help you remember the answers.

## 14. Deciding on HRT ⓘ ✎

You will only need to think about taking HRT immediately after your hysterectomy, if you are having your ovaries removed. If you haven't already gone through the menopause, you will then experience what is called a 'surgical menopause'; this can begin within twenty four hours of your hysterectomy. Whether you then choose to take HRT will depend on your own particular circumstances and attitudes. So, if you are over fifty, had already gone through the menopause and don't like the idea of taking drugs then you may decide it's not for you. Alternatively, if you're in your late thirties then you may feel that you are simply replacing the hormones you would have continued to produce naturally for some time to come.

There is no right or wrong decision to make as everyone is different and we have listed some of the pros and cons below; you may be able to add some more of your own to our list.

| Why you might | Why you might not[7] |
|---|---|
| high risk of osteoporosis | past the menopause already |
| high risk of heart disease | high risk of breast cancer |
| severe menopausal symptoms | high risk of thrombosis |
| age at hysterectomy | hysterectomy for endometriosis |

If you have a hysterectomy and your ovaries removed because you have endometriosis, then you may be advised not to take HRT for up to twelve months after your operation. This is because there is a risk that the replacement oestrogen contained in HRT will encourage a re-growth and therefore any that is still left after surgery needs to have the opportunity to die off completely.

If you do keep your ovaries after your hysterectomy, then you may find that they fail earlier than they might otherwise have done. If you start experiencing any symptoms that could be considered menopausal then you may also need to make the decision about whether or not to take HRT. Of course, there is nothing to say you have to take HRT even if you have your ovaries removed; you could choose to use more natural ways of managing any menopausal symptoms, but more about those later.

## 15. Investigate testosterone supplements ⓘ✎

If your ovaries are removed, not only will you lose oestrogen but you will also stop producing testosterone which is vital for female wellbeing as small amounts are produced throughout your menstrual cycle. If you were to go through the menopause naturally, your ovaries and adrenal glands would continue to produce testosterone for up to twelve years.

In a woman, testosterone acts directly on mood and sex drive[8]; it can also provide relief from hot flushes and night sweats. Symptoms of testosterone deficiency can include lack of libido, having no energy and depression.

If you don't want to take testosterone, then supplementing with Zinc may help, as some studies[9] have shown that impotent men taking zinc supplements improved their potency and raised their levels of testosterone to normal.

# My Notes

# Getting ready for hospital

### 16. Buying a new nightie

Yes, you are still a woman and yes, you still want and need your femininity to be recognised and acknowledged. One way to do it, even in hospital, is to treat yourself to some new nighties to celebrate finally getting back to being you again. I say nighties because pjs, although some can be very sexy, may not be as comfortable around your tummy as a nightie, and you'll probably want cotton as it's cooler. Buy two or three (you'll want another to wear when you receive all those visitors and well-wishers when you get home) and really take your time over choosing the ones that say the most about who you are going to be once the operation is over and the recovery begins.

### 17. Treat yourself to new perfume

Sexy is one thing that many of us don't feel when we have a hysterectomy; but this is one area of our lives that could benefit the most with freedom from those awful symptoms. Preparing for the 'New You' takes some planning, and treating yourself to some new perfume is one good way to start.

Choosing a scent that makes you feel good acts on all sorts of senses and can stimulate happy feelings and invoke pleasant memories for each of us. Wearing a perfume can make us feel glamorous and get us noticed; just think of the adverts on TV for perfume and what images they use to persuade us to buy them.

It is one thing, together with new night wear, that can make us feel

15

better even while we are still in hospital recovering, (but don't be tempted to spray before you have your op. or anywhere near your wound after). Some scents can even help the healing process by acting on the olfactory centres of the brain; these include lavender, myrrh, orange and ravensara.

## 18. Invaluable Arnica

Arnica homeopathic preparations are often recommended by complementary therapists for physical and emotional shock. It is thought that arnica promotes healing, helps control bleeding and reduces swelling as the herbs' active ingredients are known to have mild pain-relieving, anti-inflammatory, and antibacterial actions[10].

It is generally recommended that the homeopathic remedy is taken for three days before, and three days after, surgery according to the instructions on the container, as it is thought to it may help to cut down on recovery time after surgery. You can also use arnica cream on any bruising after your scar has healed completely.

If you do decide to take it before your operation, make sure you tell your anaesthetist as he may need to take this into account when deciding how to sedate you.

You can buy arnica from any good pharmacy. Although the homeopathic remedies are safe to use as they have been diluted many times, do not under any circumstances ingest the herb itself as it is highly poisonous.

## 19. The importance of ritual

Ritual plays an increasingly minor role in our secular society, but it can be one way of closing the door on a chapter of your life. The purpose of such a ritual is to prepare you emotionally, and perhaps mentally, for your hysterectomy by asking for help with the healing process and to acknowledge any loss you may feel. It also helps you to embrace the positive changes that the operation may be bringing into your life.

A ritual can be as simple as lighting a candle and saying a prayer; or it can involve friends that are supporting you in your recovery period. We have provided a **ritual for an operation** in the database section of The Hysterectomy Association website that you are welcome to use or adapt for your own purposes. You can find it by going to: *www.hysterectomy-association.org.uk/diaries/* - look under *resources and books* and then *complimentary health and medicine*

## 20. Buy a good book, or ten

As you won't be doing much of anything else, a good book or ten can keep you absorbed for days, and you've already made a good start by buying 101 Handy Hints for a Happy Hysterectomy! But seriously, what we're really talking about is that list of books you keep intending to read because they've been recommended by friends or the book club. Why not go to the library, visit your local book store or even check out Amazon.

Of course while you're in hospital you may not feel like holding a book up and this is when talking books can be really beneficial. Invest in a personal CD or tape player and join the local library where you'll find a huge selection of all types and titles. Yes ladies, it's time to be soothed as someone once again reads you that book at bedtime!

## 21. Start a journal ☺ ⓘ ✓

So you're having a hysterectomy? Why is that; what has life been like since you started having health problems? How has it affected your achievements, relationships and 'joie de vivre'? On the worst day you can remember describe in a sentence how you felt. How did you feel when you woke up this morning? How do you feel now? Describe what you want as an achievable goal. What's your general state of health? How's the pain and is there anything you've found that reduces the pain (lying down for example) or can you identify what caused the increase?

And suddenly you're reading your journal entry for last Monday. You decided that you were going to keep an on-going journal each day until six weeks after your hysterectomy. Even in one week you've come so far. Not only can you see you're having less pain but you also feel more in control and just look at your progress in the last week!


## 22. Buy, or borrow, a cordless 'phone

You will probably be getting lots of calls from friends and family to find out how you're doing after you get home from hospital, and one of the most frustrating things about having a hysterectomy is constantly getting up and down to answer the 'phone. Whilst it's good to exercise your abdominal muscles to help them heal, you also want to enjoy the recuperation time.

So why not do yourself a favour and buy, or borrow, a cordless 'phone, (preferably with at least two handsets so that you can have one downstairs and one upstairs). And if you don't already have one, why not consider a mobile phone as well. You can carry it around with you, and when you're out walking if you find you've overdone it then at least you can call a 'taxi' to pick you up and take you home.

But, remember this is your time to recover and you could really rebel and actually ignore the phone when it rings especially if you have an answer 'phone or subscribe to a free answering service, like BT's 1571, people can leave a message and you can get back to them later – if you want to.

## 23. Keep a scaling diary

Half the battle in getting over a hysterectomy physically, mentally and spiritually is seeing an improvement each day in the things that are important to you.  So the first task is to decide what you want to achieve.  Think about the following things and mark off right now where you feel you are.

Day: ........................./ Date: ................................. / Time: .........................

*(1 is the least/lowest you've had or done and 10 is the most/highest you've had or done)*

| ⊛ Pain | 1 | 2 | 3 | 4 | 5 | 6 | 7 | 8 | 9 | 10 |
|---|---|---|---|---|---|---|---|---|---|---|
| ⊛ Sleeping | 1 | 2 | 3 | 4 | 5 | 6 | 7 | 8 | 9 | 10 |
| ⊛ Mood | 1 | 2 | 3 | 4 | 5 | 6 | 7 | 8 | 9 | 10 |
| ⊛ Tiredness | 1 | 2 | 3 | 4 | 5 | 6 | 7 | 8 | 9 | 10 |
| ⊛ Exercise/Walking | 1 | 2 | 3 | 4 | 5 | 6 | 7 | 8 | 9 | 10 |
| Comments: | | | | | | | | | | |

At the end of this book is a page you can use as a template for your own scaling diary or you can make your own up before you go into hospital.  For the first week or two you could fill it in two or three times a day as this will help you see patterns emerge.  Use this together with your journal and within a couple of weeks you'll be able to see how much you're improving;

small baby steps towards it at first, and then big giant leaps later on.


## 24. Cultivate calm and happiness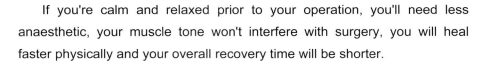

If you're calm and relaxed prior to your operation, you'll need less anaesthetic, your muscle tone won't interfere with surgery, you will heal faster physically and your overall recovery time will be shorter.

> *Sounds good, you'll have some of that?*
> *So how do you achieve it?*


First of all you've got to be convinced in your own mind that a hysterectomy is right for you and that you're in control. You need to be able to visualise in vivid detail how much better your life will be post recovery.

Make a list on one side of a page in your journal about how much your health problems have held you back and affected your life and relationships.

Now, on the other side write down how you will use the post-recovery benefits when released from those drawbacks. And when you are describing the benefits, use enough detail to make it real for you, as if you're experiencing it now. Then, whenever you feel frightened, are feeling pain or discomfort or just feeling down, revisit your list and relive the destinations that you set out on this journey to achieve, and give yourself some serious lovin', because you're one big brave girl!


## 25. Time to talk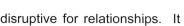

The time before a hysterectomy can be disruptive for relationships. It can seem as if a slice of life has been removed. Many women on the helpline describe how their work and leisure time has had to accommodate detailed planning on every single thing for a week or two each month, twelve times a year. Your mood may have swung all over the place, tears one minute, incandescent rage the next, and all your closest relationships have also had to cope with this. Your hysterectomy may well be opening up a whole new life and its time to talk about what you want this to be like.

Do you and your partner communicate well? Do they know of your hopes and fears about your hysterectomy, do you know of theirs? A non-confrontational way of talking about how you view life after hysterectomy is to play a needs and expectations game where you each write down what you believe the other persons needs (can't do without) and expectations (would like to have) about your hysterectomy are. When you've written them down, swap your lists and use the insights as way of addressing all those expectations. This can actually open up a new world of relating by removing previous blocks and misconceptions. Enjoy laughing at areas where you both made assumptions about each other and use your new found knowledge to create a closer relationship for the future.

## 26. Monitoring oestrogen levels for long term health

If you have a hysterectomy that removes your ovaries, you will start the menopause immediately regardless of your age (unless you have already had it); this is called a surgical menopause. However, if your ovaries are left in place, you have a fifty percent chance of them failing within five years of surgery and going into the menopause early. It can be helpful in this case to have your blood oestrogen levels measured before your hysterectomy takes place, as this gives your GP something to compare future results against.

Oestrogen levels can be measured with a simple blood test, and several may be taken over the course of your cycle prior to surgery to get a good baseline result. Falling levels of oestrogen in your blood tests after your hysterectomy can be a good indicator that your ovaries are failing, at which point you can then make a decision about how you will navigate through the menopause.

### 27. Don't try to be Superwoman

Most of us think we're superwoman; not only do we get the children up and off to school, we have a full time job, make sure everyone eats regularly and is wearing clean knickers (just in case they get run over). The problem with a hysterectomy is that the image we have of ourselves being superwoman takes a bit of a battering and about time too!

Let's face it, the men (or others) in our lives are perfectly capable of cooking a meal, doing the grocery shopping and ironing the washing; our problem is that we think they don't do it right, so we have to do it 'properly'.

But now is the time to let the standards slip a little and to accept with gracious thanks all the efforts that are made by the men, women and children around us that help to make our recovery just that little bit easier.

If your partner doesn't know one end of a wash cycle from another, explain it to him, show him and then get him to do it; then write out instructions beginning with sorting the laundry into the right piles. If they don't know what to buy in the weekly shop, make it easy and give them a list of the things you buy every week and you never know some welcome little treats might come home as well.

The advantage of all this preparation, of course, is that when you are back on your feet again, there can be no more excuses to avoid sharing the household tasks!

An even bigger bonus is that when your significant other understands that stacking the dishwasher, loading the washing machine and doing the ironing is making such a difference to your recovery, they might be getting more positive strokes from you than they've had all day and that's got to be good for the relationship.

## 28. Progesterone

Progesterone (progestin) is used by the female body to help maintain pregnancy, protect against the 'build-up' effect of oestrogen which is linked to womb and breast cancer and prevent ovulation taking place in the second half of the menstrual cycle.

After the menopause the production of progesterone stops and if you have a hysterectomy that removes the ovaries then your progesterone production will stop as well.

There is some research which suggests that progestins have a positive influence on bone, heart, brain and other tissues and that they may be beneficial for women that cannot take oestrogen[11]. However, other research suggests that higher levels of progesterone may be a risk factor in breast cancer[12].

If you feel that progesterone might be beneficial then it could be worth considering the herbal supplements Dong Quai and Black Cohosh as they are considered by complementary therapists to have similar effects.

## 29. Managing Child Care ✍ ✓

Do you still have young or school age children?  If so managing child care is more than just arranging for someone to pick them up from school or look after them in the holidays.  How about finding out about the local after school clubs so that your partner, parents or friends can collect them after work and why not talk to other parents about how to manage the school run, ask for help - the worst they can say is No.

You will also need to think about the needs of your younger children as you won't be able to pick them up for a few weeks, and they won't be able to jump on top of you. Maybe some of the activities you always do together, such as swimming might need to stop for a while; but don't just stop them on the day you come out of hospital though. It is important that you explain to *all* of your family what your hysterectomy will mean for you, and how it will affect them, well before the day of the operation so that they can be prepared as well.

## 30. Invest in a recovery pillow ☺✔

It could be a favourite cushion from home, or a comfortable pillow from your bed; you could even go out and buy a special one, just to cuddle while you're not well.

Either way, you'll use it most days after your operation for many different things. It'll be the most fantastic comfort blanket when you feel sad or fed-up, and it's something comfy to rest your feet on when you've had your daily dose of walking. You can cuddle it to your tummy when you want to laugh or cough as it will support your aching muscles. You'll be able to lie on your side with it stuffed under your tummy, providing just enough support until you get used to the very strange shifting and pulling feeling. Finally, stuffed between you and the seat belt, it will stop it rubbing against the wound when you're a passenger in the car again. So ladies, meet Pillow, your new best friend!

## 31. Get a new hairstyle

Having a new hairstyle is one of the easiest ways to help you feel better in the short term while recovering from your operation. Not only will you know you look good, but getting one that is easy to look after will mean that you don't have to worry too much about hair gels, sprays and styling.

One thing you won't want to do is lift your arms up for long periods of time for drying as this will pull on any scar and your traumatised tummy muscles. Personally, I'd go for something young and funky; you definitely won't look, or feel, your years when you see yourself in the mirror. To get the perfect hairstyle, book in a long appointment with your favourite hairstylist and talk over with them what suits the shape of your face and the image you would like. One thing's for sure, you won't regret it afterwards and there does seem to be a strong link between looking good and feeling better.


## 32. Give blood

For the vast majority of women, their hysterectomy operation goes without a hitch. However, for the occasional few there may be problems, which could result in a serious loss of blood. If you have an unusual blood type it may be worth discussing with your GP and/or gynaecologist whether it is possible to make a donation of blood, specifically for use in the event of a problem. In the event that your blood isn't needed, it could then be used in the general blood bank.

As well as making a donation of blood, having a really good blood count is important for your long term recovery and to help prevent anaemia. With this in mind, it is probably worth increasing your intake of green leafy vegetables, which are a good source of iron, as well as other strongly pigmented foods such as carrots and peppers, which contain the vitamin A and calcium, needed to absorb any iron supplements you may be given.

When you've had your operation it may be a good idea to ask for a blood count to be done (if they don't do one as a matter of course), just to check that your iron levels are up to scratch.

# So now you're in the hospital

## 33. Water, the greatest healer

Around fifty-five to sixty percent of our bodies are made up of water, in fact the brain is more than seventy percent water by weight, and if it dips below its critical level you will feel listless, dull and very light headed.  It is no wonder then that we need a lot just to manage our daily lives.

After the operation you will be dehydrated and your body will be trying to rid itself of toxins, such as the anaesthetics, and you may be at risk of developing a urinary tract infection because of the catheter that's been inserted.

However, by taking lots of liquids, especially plain water, you will be giving your body the best chance of avoiding any of these problems.  As well as flushing the body out, it will also help to keep your stools soft, so that they are easier to pass and it will help you go to the loo regularly as well.

The recommended intake is around one and a half to two litres per day. This can be in plain water, weak teas, herbal and fruit teas, milk, fruit juice and squash and you can tell when you're drinking enough, because your urine will be almost colourless.

## 34. Relaxation and meditation

There is no doubt about it, being calm and relaxed before any operation is definitely the best approach; being stressed and fearful may increase the risk of any side effects or other problems during your hysterectomy or later recovery.

There are many ways to achieve a calm mind before surgery, but one of the best is to use a tape or CD specifically designed to help you relax.

I would recommend using the CD or tape for a week or so before your hysterectomy, either before bedtime or at some other quiet point in the day. And once you return from hospital, it is going to be very helpful for maintaining a relaxed state of mind while your body takes over the job of getting you fit and well again.

## 35. Get your bowels moving

Dehydration and pain are the most common reasons why women have problems getting back into a regular bowel rhythm after a hysterectomy. Both can prevent the bowel from opening properly, particularly when the expectation of pain is high. It is likely, though, that you won't be allowed to leave hospital until you have had at least one bowel movement.

Drinking lots of water and other weak fluids, as well as warm water and lemon juice first thing in the morning will help enormously. A gentle laxative or some natural fibre added to your breakfast cereal will probably deal with the most stubborn cases.

Once you're at home, gently massaging your abodomen in a clockwise direction, being careful not to rub too hard, will encourage the normal motion of the bowel and by taking supplements such as fish and olive oils, you can help to keep the stools soft so that they don't become dry, hard and too painful to pass.

Of course, plenty of fibrous fruit and vegetables will be a great addition to your diet; so why not increase your intake even before surgery.

## 36. How do I get out of bed?

It's amazing how many of the abdominal muscles you use doing things we all take for granted such as getting out of bed. After a hysterectomy it can become a real effort and will take a lot of thinking about in order to achieve it.

This way seems to work for most women. Shuffle over to within about twelve inches of the side of the bed you would like to get out of; pull your knees up so your heels are against your bottom and slowly turn over on your side facing the edge of the bed. Slowly, manoeuvre your knees and legs over the side of the bed and allow them to act as a counterweight as you push up with your arms until you are sitting upright on the side.

If you simply want to sit up in bed, pull your heels under your bottom and push hard into the mattress with your hands and feet to prevent using your abdominal muscles to pull you up. Incidentally this way of getting out of bed is also really good if you ever suffer from a bad back!

## 37. Acknowledging your femininity

So you've got the special nightie and the new perfume and even the hairstyle. Looking good makes you feel good and this is even more true when you're recovering from surgery; it gives you an incentive to get up and try things and to keep doing a little extra each day until you feel more like your old self again.

Let's face it, there are so many opportunities just knocking on the door once your recovery is over and done with. Just imagine the knickers you can buy, now that they haven't got to be stuffed with multiple pads and you don't have to wear them several sizes too large to accommodate the fibroids or bloating.

Have you thought about what you can wear now that floaty skirts, summer dresses and beautiful cream linen trousers are back in the frame again? Looking forward to doing those things you couldn't do before helps you remember that you're still a sexy, wonderful and beautiful woman.

## 38. Affirmations for health

Having confidence in your own ability to help yourself heal is one of the keys to active wellness. A lot of how well you feel is governed by your mood and attitude to life in general; if you expect things to go well and believe that you are going to be healthy and happy in the future, then the chances are that this is what you'll get.

To help get these positive feelings working for your benefit, you are going to devise your own affirmation. The key to affirmations is repetition; if you say them regularly and with conviction then you will be retraining your mind to think in this new and positive way. So, think about what you want to include; will it be no pain and freedom from the restrictions on your lifestyle, the new image that you will have or the energy you can expect?

Make your words and phrases fit with who you are, and make sure you keep it very much in the present. If you put it into the future then it will remain in the future. So you might say something like "I'm feeling full of energy and I have no pain". At first it may feel a bit false, but the more you say it, the more you will feel it, so please do persevere.

As well as saying your own affirmations, why not ask your family and friends to keep you in their thoughts and send you a healing prayer or thought. Knowing that people are thinking of you and wishing you the very best, makes a positive statement about how much others value your presence in their life, and this makes you feel even better!

## 39. Peppermint and other teas

One of the most uncomfortable side-effects of gynaecological surgery is wind, with many women rating it amongst the top three stressors. While a few hospitals now make peppermint tea or cordial available as a matter of course, unless yours is definitely one of them; take your own. Not only is it good for wind, it's also good for the digestion, contains no caffeine, isn't a diuretic and, when it's combined with honey, a natural sleep promoter.

And it's not the only tea with therapeutic properties by a long chalk. Green Tea is a decongestant, anti-inflammatory, aids absorption of vitamins and boosts the immune system. Red Bush tea brightens you up, is low in caffeine and is a great for the digestive tract; while Siberian Ginseng tea restores immediate, and long term, energy supplies, overcomes stress and fatigue and helps to maintain blood sugar levels. Finally, Oolong Tea is great for the digestion, is a natural stimulant and boosts positive mood.

## 40. Help yourself prevent thrombosis

It is highly likely that after surgery you will be discovered wearing some highly appealing, and very sexy, white surgical compression stockings! These are put on before, or during, your hysterectomy to help prevent blood clots from forming in the deep veins of the legs during the operation and later while you are spending much of your time in bed resting. DVT (deep vein thrombosis) is comparatively rare and affects around only one or two people in every 1000.

If you do get a DVT, then there are two possible complications that may occur; pulmonary embolus (a blood clot which travels to the lung) or post thrombotic syndrome (persistent calf symptoms). For these reasons it is advisable to make sure that you do any exercises given to you by physiotherapy staff in the hospital.

You can also help to prevent any problems by ensuring you drink plenty of water, which helps your circulation, and by walking as far as you can as soon after your hysterectomy as possible. The muscles in the lower legs act like little pumps and as you walk they help to keep the blood circulating and prevent it from forming clots. Raising the level of your feet on pillows or cushions whenever you are resting will also take the pressure off your calf veins. The highest incidence of pulmonary embolus occurs within twenty four hours after your hysterectomy, although they can happen up to three weeks later, so it is important to continue doing the exercises, the walking and keeping your legs raised during rest times, even when you get home.

## 41. Managing pain (i) ✍

Pain is the body's way of telling us something is wrong and as we all know, it can range from simple discomfort to agony. We will all feel it differently though, as we don't have the same pain threshold. After a hysterectomy, your pain will be managed in two ways. Initially, you will have a PCA (patient controlled analgesia) fitted, which will probably contain morphine. This means that you'll be in control of your pain medication. To deliver a shot, you simply press the button. The PCA device contains a built in timer, so you can't overdose yourself. Your PCA will be removed sometime within the first twenty four to forty eight hours.

After your PCA device has been removed, you will be given regular painkillers for surgical pain depending on how much pain you are in.

Once you're at home, Ibuprofen and Paracetamol will probably be advised, although you may feel you need something stronger, which your GP can prescribe. As you progress through your recovery, your need for pain control will become less.

If, once you get home, you don't like the idea of taking too many tablets then you could consider combining them with a more natural approach, such as acupuncture or acupressure. Both operate on the principle of body 'trigger points' where applying a needle or finger pressure to a specific point will relieve pain. They can also stimulate the body to produce more endorphins (the body's natural pain relievers).

Visualising the natural healing process going on within your body is also very therapeutic, and it can help manage pain levels. Why not imagine you've packed the area in pain with ice, and gradually feel it freezing.

Don't forget to keep monitoring your levels of pain in your scaling diary. Not only will this show you how far you've come, but it can help you to spot any potential problems.

### 42. So just what does happen in hospital?

On **day one**, after your surgery, you will probably feel aches and pains all over your body, have a stiff-neck and abdominal pain (this can continue for several days). You will probably find that you are attached to patient controlled analgesia, do use it, you can't overdose. You will probably be catheterised so you don't have to worry about going to the loo to pass urine and you will probably be attached to a saline drip to compensate for dehydration. Drink as much as possible as the more you drink, the sooner the drip will be removed. Don't plan any visits except from your nearest and dearest as you will be drifting in and out of sleep and you won't want to feel responsible for maintaining a conversation.

On **day two**, you will probably have the catheter removed, and you will be encouraged to get up and walk to the loo, with some support. Once you're over the wobbles, try and walk as much as possible, it won't be far, just around the bed or the ward at first, but the more you do, the better you will feel. If you do have visitors encourage them to keep it brief and bring some lovely flowers. You may also have some discharge or slight bleeding, this is perfectly normal. The physiotherapists may come to show you some simple exercises to help prevent DVT, if they didn't do it before your operation.

On **day three**, have a warm and gentle shower, you'll feel so much better, but try and keep your dressing and the wound dry. By now you should be thinking about opening your bowels, if this doesn't happen, then you could ask for a mild laxative as well drinking as much warm water as possible. You could also expect to have a blood count done, to check you aren't anaemic. You may be feeling quite low and weepy and once again this is perfectly normal.

On **day four** or five, you could be having any staples removed.

By **day five**, if all has gone well, and depending on the hospital policies, you will probably be well enough to join the escape committee and go home to start your recovery proper. Don't forget to pack something loose and comfortable to wear for the drive home; your recovery pillow, tucked inside the seat belt will prevent any rubbing or chaffing against any wound you have.

These are the average times for most women, but your hospital may be different, so do make sure you collect any leaflets or information packs.

# 43. Make up a hospital basket

Let's face it, being in hospital is not going to be the most exciting time of your life and although you will be meeting other women to talk to, you will probably want a few other things to do on the few days you're going to be in.

Why not make up a basket to take in with you that contains a book, magazine, a puzzle book, pens, notelets, your personal CD player or tape player as well as some music and audio books to listen to. You could also take in your hysterectomy journal and scaling diary so that you can monitor your own progress. The odd relaxation tape or CD can work wonders to quell the nerves before your operation; and to help send you off to sleep after. And what about including peppermint tea bags, mineral water and juice to ensure you're drinking enough fluids.

Then there's the food. Why not take in a treat or two, perhaps some chocolate, biscuits or fruit. And remember you can share them all with your new friends on the ward as there's nothing quite like a gossip about operations over a choccie biscuit or two!

# My Notes

# Recovery Time

## 44. Inner cleansing drink

Pineapple is high in the enzyme bromelain which is a natural anti-inflammatory and it encourages healing. Limes are full of Vitamin C, as is apple juice and they are both full of anti-oxidants.

---

- 1 carton live yoghurt
- 1 small can unsweetened pineapple chunks
- 1 small bottle of freshly pressed apple juice
- Juice of 1 lime
- Drizzle of honey to taste (if required)
- Handful of ice to cool it all down.

Pop it all in a blender and crush it all into a really thick smooth drink, decorate with a slice of lime, if you fancy, and sip it over the course of an hour.

---

## 45. Pelvic floor exercises

The pelvic floor muscles are two groups of muscles situated around the urethra, vagina and anus. They provide support to your womb, bladder and bowel. After your womb is removed, the other organs will shift around the abdomen and there may be a small risk of prolapse later in life.

Pelvic floor exercises (Kegel exercises) are useful to help prevent prolapse and urinary incontinence and they also tone up the vagina as well.

They consist of alternately contracting and relaxing the pubococcygeous muscle, which is the one that controls your urine flow. The simplest way to do the exercise is to locate the muscle by trying to stop the flow of urine the next time you go to the loo. Once you have identified where the muscle is and what it feel like to contract it you can do the following exercise whenever and wherever you want to.

Pull the muscles up for a count of five and then relax. Repeat this process about ten times, two or three times, a day.

## 46. The value of walking

One of the easiest ways to get the exercise you need after your hysterectomy is to walk. Walking helps improve your circulation, gets the bowel moving and guards against deep vein thrombosis. It will calm your mind, help you to relax and just thirty minutes a day of brisk walking when you are fully recovered will mean your heart remains healthy, as well as keeping the weight off.

You will probably be encouraged to walk the day after surgery and may be advised to increase the distance a little every day remembering to try and walk upright as you don't want to strain your back. Why not keep a note in your journal of how far you walk everyday; remember that every step around the house counts too. Perhaps you could persuade someone to get you a pedometer so that you can accurately measure how far you actually walk; it will probably be further than you think.

## 47. Water retention

Because you aren't doing as much as usual, water retention can be a common symptom after a hysterectomy and it can also be a side effect of some forms of hormone replacement therapy. It appears as swelling in the ankles and lower legs or in the tummy area and can be very uncomfortable as well as making you feel very self conscious. In some cases it can be so bad that you have problems getting shoes on your feet or rings on your fingers.

Despite your natural inclination not to drink too much, actually increasing your water intake to around one and half to two litres a day can help as it means your body isn't holding onto fluids because it feels dehydrated. As well as increasing the amount of water you drink, limiting the amount of salt you eat and increasing the distances and frequency of walking are all beneficial; walking helps because the muscles at the bottom of the legs act a little like pumps that get blood and lymph fluids circulating.

Dandelion and Parsley supplements are both natural diuretics and you could also try drinking Fennel tea. Adding Fennel oil to a warm bath will have a similar effect or why not massage your body, particularly your legs, with Fennel diluted in carrier oil?

## 48. Aloe vera and cats claw

So what's a Roman soldier got to do with your hysterectomy? Well, about 3000 years ago, seriously wounded soldiers were sent to an island colonised by plants with spiky, rubbery leaves. They found that by drinking the juice and by rubbing a freshly broken leaf on a wound, they healed twice as quickly as their colleagues.

Nowadays, we also appreciate the many other virtues of one of nature's most powerful healers, both internal and external.

Many conditions are reputed to respond to Aloe Vera including Candida, chronic fatigue, low immune system, ulcers, viral infections, arthritis, colds and digestive tract problems including irritable bowel syndrome. Externally, Aloe Vera preparations are available to ease aches and pains.

Cat's Claw (so named for its appearance) is possibly one of the world's most important herbal discoveries. From the Peruvian rain forest, this herb works at many levels within the body, its reported therapeutic benefits[13] are linked to Candida and cancer, allergies, intestinal disorders, depression and HIV. Apparently, when it's used in conjunction with Aloe Vera, the effects can be amazing. However, as with all complementary therapies, check their use with your GP beforehand, especially if you are taking other medication, and do make sure you follow the manufacturer's instructions.

### 49. Flower power

The sight and smell of flowers is very uplifting and their scent can be very heady encouraging emotional responses in us that encourage our body to release 'feel good' hormones. As well as being given flowers, you can also imagine them in a relaxation exercise.

Close your eyes and breathe deeply. Imagine a beautiful bud, slowly it unfurls and becomes a beautiful flower in full bloom, just relax looking at the flower in your minds eye and remember that this is what you are, a flower that is coming into full bloom.

The flowers that you choose for your relaxation exercise also have potent meanings, for instance the Azalea is the Chinese symbol of womanhood and the chrysanthemum means cheerfulness, optimism, rest and truth. The Daffodil is associated with re-birth and new beginnings and Yarrow is for healing.

## 50. Comfy loose clothes 😊 ✎ ✔

After you've come home from hospital, you should stay in your night clothes as much as possible for a week or two. Not only will this be one less thing to worry about, but it will also help other people around you remember that you are recovering from a major operation, and therefore not to expect too much from you.

As you get back to feeling more like your old self, then you will want to be dressed again, especially for walking up and down the road; no guesses about what might happen if you go out in just your new nighty!

Loose clothes, such as princess line dresses that fall from just below the bust, tracksuit bottoms, elasticated and drawstring skirts and trousers, whilst not the most fashionable of items will take the strain off your tummy muscles and will allow any wound you may have to breathe and heal as naturally as possible. Loose and full tops worn over what's on the bottom will help you disguise the elastic and cord ties that you're using just now. T-shirts or tops in bright colours will also distract other peoples' eyes from your bottom half and will have the added benefit of cheering you up as well. Try to avoid tights and other close fitting underwear, and stick to socks when you need to put something on your feet.

## 51. Create a relax corner 😊 ✔

Take care of yourself and make sure that you don't have to get up and down too frequently by creating a cosy corner just for you in your sitting room. With a table and a big basket, you can keep your books, magazines, telephone, bottled water and a thermos of tea handy. Don't forget remote controls for things like the stereo and TV. You can also keep your personal stereo handy so that you can use your relaxation tapes, and what about your recovery pillow, a warm blanket and hot water bottle if you feel the cold.

You will need a comfortable chair or sofa with lots of soft cushions and a big footstool, or low table piled with cushions, to put your feet up on. If it is summer and the weather is good, why not create it in the garden for the day.

Don't forget to let everyone in the house know that this is your special, personal space to be used only by you while you're recovering.

## 52. Helpful supplements

There is no doubt about it, having surgery is a testing time for your body and some extra help would be very much appreciated.

For instance, Vitamin C is used by the body for tissue repair and growth as well as for healing wounds, but the body can't retain it and so it needs to be replenished daily. Vitamin E is also good for healing as it promotes the production of new blood cells. Selenium is a key antioxidant that works with Vitamin E to protect our cells from free radicals and improves immunity; it is also an anti-inflammatory and is thought to help with menopausal symptoms. Zinc is one of the most important trace minerals for our bodies as it has a major part to play in maintenance of body tissue and our immune system. It is also called the 'healing mineral' as it speeds up the healing process.

If you are thinking about supplementing, do check with your GP that there will be no adverse reactions to any other drugs you're taking. The easiest way to take any of these healing helpers is in a good quality multi-vitamin and mineral supplement.

## 53. Make a healing smoothie

If you don't fancy taking even more tablets, why not try our recipe for a healing smoothie; it's tasty and full of Vitamin C, Vitamin E and Selenium.

> ⊛ 1 small bottle/cup of freshly squeezed orange juice
>
> ⊛ Handful of strawberries (fresh or frozen)
>
> ⊛ Large teaspoon of wheat germ
>
> Whizz them all together in the blender and pour into a large glass, decorate with fresh mint, if you feel like it.   Then sit down, relax and enjoy the moment.

## 54. Perfect relaxation

Entering a more relaxed state will help to calm any physical tension so that you are able to be more responsive to creative, healing and positive thoughts.   How do you normally relax?  Some people can get lost in music, others achieve inner peace in a garden, while yet more may be in a world of their own when dancing.

A creative, yet simple way of relaxing, is using visualisation. Think of a place or time when you were really happy and relaxed. It might have been on a beach or in a wood; it could be that perfect afternoon when you planted those two apple trees, or that night on the dance floor when free expression and the music took over.   Whatever you choose, you need to be able to recreate it vividly in your minds eye.

Settle down somewhere comfortable, become aware of your breathing, consciously taking slightly longer to breathe out.   Empty your mind of all your day to day concerns and go back to your own special time and place. Play it back to yourself, complete with sound, smells, temperature, people and feelings. Experience the bliss and enjoy it to the full; feel good about yourself, smile inside and feel the love.

While you were away in your imagination, your breathing and heart will have slowed down; your brain was releasing pleasure hormones and your immune system was being pumped up with energy, your muscles were relaxed. Now you're back; how do you feel?

## 55. Banish the sweats naturally ✍

Hot flushes and night sweats are a major symptom of the menopause which, for some women, can be unbearable and very disruptive whilst others will barely notice them and their effects. They can make you feel very self conscious even though they often aren't detectable to anyone else.

Research has shown that a combination of Vitamin C and Bioflavonoids[14] are very effective at controlling hot flushes, and the recommended dose is between one to three grams per day. In addition Vitamin E seems to have a positive effect on these symptoms.

Herbal remedies can also be very helpful and the American Indians have used Black Cohosh effectively for centuries. It has been shown to be effective in balancing female hormones as well relieving menopausal symptoms[15]. Yarrow has also been used to lower body temperature whilst Vitex agnus Castus is considered one of the most potent remedies because it stimulates and balances the pituitary gland which, in turn, controls and balances our hormones: it's also good for reducing hot flushes[16].

Korean red ginseng can also help with any depression you may feel. And, increasing phyto-nutrients through fruit and vegetables can help to balance the body. Omega 3 fatty acids may help prevent post-menopausal osteoporosis, breast cancer and cardio-vascular disease.

Flavonoids, such as hesperidin from Citrus fruits, when combined with Vitamin C, have been shown to relieve hot flushes. And finally, aromatherapy massage, perhaps using sage, chamomile and lavender; seems to help some menopausal symptoms – seems like an excellent reason to indulge!

## 56. Ten things you must NOT do (for at least four to six weeks)

No vacuuming

No lifting (anything more than a half full kettle)

No sex (until the top of your vagina has healed)

No driving

No bending, unless you use your knees and keep your back straight

No stretching to get things off a high shelf

No bed making

No gardening

No stacking or unstacking the dishwasher and washing machine

Definitely no skateboarding!

At the end of this book are some pages with a list which you can photocopy and put on a convenient cupboard or wall to tell the whole family what you can, and CAN'T do, while you are recovering.

## 57. The joy of massage

Massage is one of the nicest ways to help your body heal itself, while giving yourself a good pampering at the same time. You don't necessarily have to go to a professional as it is possible to self massage, particularly for bloating, dispelling wind and general relaxation. The kneading, pummelling, stroking and rubbing of massage relieves muscle tension and triggers the release of endorphins. At the same time, most forms of massage also act on the lymphatic system, helping to remove toxins from the body.

When you're ready to think about having sex with your partner again, massage can be one way of easing you both into it by helping to relax the muscles that you might tense in anticipation of experiencing the same pain you may have had before your hysterectomy.

And, aromatherapy massage can be beneficial for managing the pain of any urinary tract infections you may have, particularly by massaging rosemary oil diluted in a carrier oil into your legs. If you find yourself suffering from water retention, then a lower back and abdominal massage, by your partner, with carrier oil and either grapefruit, carrot seed or juniper oil may help to ease the discomfort.

## 58. Relaxing reflexology

Reflexology is a wonderful technique as it uses nothing more than strategically placed finger pressure to relieve stress and other health problems. Reflexologists say that the technique relieves tension, improves circulation and enhances nerve function. The heel area of your feet relates to the pelvic area and the points around the outside of the ankle are associated with female reproductive organs in particular. Gentle massage of this area could help to stimulate the body's natural healing processes, but be careful as it might be quite painful to touch too firmly. Another useful point to know about is the web of skin between the thumb and forefinger, which when gently rubbed can help to ease a tension headache.

## 59. A little live yoghurt goes a long way

After any major surgery, your body is going to be in crisis and finding ways to overcome this is the key to getting back on your feet as quickly as possible. One way of supporting your system, after a diet of anaesthetics, pain killers and antibiotics, is by taking live yoghurt on a daily basis. Lactobacillus acidophilus, which is one of the main constituents of live yoghurt, has been found to have a positive effect in maintaining, or regaining, the body's natural pH level as well as increasing our body's levels of 'good' bacteria[17]. Of course, when choosing your brand of live yoghurt, do make sure that you get one without added sugar as that may undo some of the benefits you would otherwise see.

## 60. Invest in a few chick flicks !

Once you get out of hospital you're not going to be able to do very much, so why not take the opportunity to borrow, rent, or buy, all those films you've said you wanted to watch in the past. Nothing too stressful mind, because you won't want to tense your tummy muscles too much, but a little laughter (with your handy recovery pillow at hand) could be just what the doctor ordered.

What about joining the local library as they often have CD's, DVD's and videos these days, and you can ask your partner, a friend or relative to change them for you when you can't get there for yourself.  You could even rent DVD's online from Amazon if you have access to the internet at home; they send them to you through the post.

And if you think you might have a problem expressing any emotions that come up after your hysterectomy then an old fashioned weepy is a good excuse to cry without needing to offer any explanations to anyone else.

## 61. Simple abundance

It is easy when we're recovering from a major operation to forget to be thankful for everything that is actually going right in our lives, from living in the UK where we can access medical care reasonably easily, free of charge (most of the time) and where many of us can take time off from our daily lives to get on with the task of getting better.

Just spending time 'being' is one of the most important things you can do to aid your recovery and appreciating all the little 'gifts' that come your way can be very therapeutic.  In your journal why not keep a Simple Abundance record as well, by listing four or five things about the day that were good and that you really appreciated.  It might be as simple as being able to sit in the garden for the afternoon with your book, having your partner do all the clothes washing, a special visit from family and friends, or someone doing the shopping for you.  It doesn't have to be much, but it's surprising how concentrating on the good things, make the bad seem less significant somehow.

## 62. Buy a support cushion 😊

After a hysterectomy you're going to be doing quite a lot of sitting and reclining and a good support cushion can be a real investment. These V shaped cushions, which are available from most bed linen stockists, help to keep your back, neck and shoulders well supported and can be used on chairs, sofa's and beds. You could even take it into hospital with you for maximum comfort during your stay.

## 63. Managing painful wind 😊 ✔

There is no doubt that wind is going to be one of the biggest pains in the backside you are going to experience after your hysterectomy! But there are several tried and tested methods of getting rid of it, just pick the one that appeals most to you.

⊛ Drinking peppermint tea or cordial
⊛ Gently rubbing your tummy in a clockwise direction
⊛ Taking charcoal tablets
⊛ Drinking anything slightly gassy, like mineral or soda water
⊛ Chew chewing gum
⊛ Walking

## 64. Award yourself recovery treats ❗

Why not get used to rewarding yourself every time you do something that helps your recovery. Let's say you walk a hundred metres or drink your target amount of water, then why not give yourself a treat? You could get lost in a novel or a film, have some hot chocolate, make a smoothie, visit a friend, paint a picture, write a poem, buy some flowers and put them where you spend most time or even have an aromatic bath (after your wound has healed of course).

You can make a list of all your Favourite Things (Oh yes, I forgot - singing like Julie Andrews!) and choose the reward that gives you most pleasure.

With each reward tell yourself how much you deserve it, you're special and you're doing the very best that you can for your recovery right now.

## 65. Getting some tummy support

After your hysterectomy you will probably want to avoid activities that could actually help your tummy muscles recover. Deep breathing, coughing, laughing and walking upright can all seem frightening because you expect to feel pain.

You will probably want to hunch over every time you try any of these but it is important to straighten up, as good posture promotes healing by creating just enough tension in the abdominal muscles to strengthen them without hurting your wound. Hunching over, on the other hand, will cause you to lose your balance, discourage you from breathing deeply and it may even strain your back. You may be shown how to hold your recovery pillow over your wound to help to keep the muscles firm, but there is a limit to how much you may want to take Pillow out with you when taking your daily walk! When you get home from your hysterectomy, you might find a tummy support band useful as it will give gentle support to the whole abdominal region, and your back, while you get your confidence back.

## 66. Balancing hormones naturally

Our bodies need hormones to help regulate their normal functions and after having a hysterectomy that removes your ovaries the most important ones to consider are oestrogen, testosterone and progesterone. You may have decided that you don't want to, or can't, take hormone replacement therapy and will be thinking about natural alternatives to HRT.

The menopause is an entirely natural cycle of life that all women will go through and there are now many natural remedies available that are helpful for troublesome night sweats and hot flushes.

Some of the most important to look out for are phyto-oestrogens, which can be found in a wide variety of foods such as Soya and Linseeds. You can buy Burgen bread from your local supermarket, or what about making your very own menopause cake, both of which provide a good source of phyto-oestrogens.

However, as with HRT, you may find that it takes a while and a few false starts before finding the best combination for you, so don't give up and keep on trying. If you would like more information about how to manage the menopause naturally, then 'The New Alternatives to HRT' by Marilyn Glenville is just about the best book available.

## 67. Bach flower remedies

Dr Edward Bach devised thirty eight homoeopathically prepared plant and flower based remedies to treat a variety of feelings and emotions. The one you may be most familiar with is Rescue Remedy, which is used to treat shock, including shock to the physical body (so it might be useful to take a bottle into hospital with you). Others that may be supportive after a hysterectomy are Mimulus which treats the fear of known things, such as fear relating to the operation itself or of not being able to cope afterwards. Star of Bethlehem can also be used to deal with the after effects of shock, Oak is good for those who are exhausted but are struggling to carry on. Gorse is a great support if you have overwhelming despondency and despair and Olive is useful for dealing with a lack of energy. When you do have to face going back to work, use Hornbeam; it's good for that 'Monday morning feeling'.

## 68. Am I still a woman?

Our body image is central to how we see ourselves in the world and for some women this will be a huge question, whilst for others it will matter not a jot. There is no right or wrong way to feel as each is as valid and real as the other. But being prepared by asking this question before your hysterectomy will help those affected badly to make sense of any loss and to begin the process of recovering a new understanding of your womanhood.

One woman I've spoken to has said that she coped by realising that the surgery had simply removed the nursery but left the playpen! Of course this may only apply to those women who have had children and feel their family is complete. For those of us that didn't, the emotions may be very different.

We each need to ask ourselves what it is that makes us uniquely feminine. Writing these thoughts and emotions down in your hysterectomy journal will enable you to process the thoughts and then work out how to deal with them. The reality of course is that you are still, and always will be, a woman, whether you have had a hysterectomy or not.

If you are troubled by your feelings after your hysterectomy, then you may find our e-book *'Losing the Woman Within'* very helpful. Part story, part information it is written by someone who has been there and who has experienced the full range of emotions after her hysterectomy.

## 69. Listen to your body ⓘ ✍ ✔

You are the expert on your body.  Your body is healthy in its natural state.  Provide it with enough sleep, a good diet and plenty of water and it will respond by giving you the energy you need to function every day.

However, now you've had a hysterectomy your body needs to let you know how best to help it back to health.  And it's here that, providing you listen to your body, pain can be a positive asset in the healing process.  So for the first few weeks after your operation, mark in your scaling diary the levels of pain you are feeling and at what times of the day.  You can also write in the notes section the reason you think it might be worse than usual.

## 70. Bleeding and discharge ☺ ⓘ

Many women complain about having bleeding and discharge for a few weeks after having a hysterectomy.  It is perfectly normal for this to happen and it can last from several days to several weeks.  It usually becomes darker and turns into spotting as time goes on, but it can also be bright red.

The majority of post operative bleeding will be due to the normal healing process, the vagina expelling any clotted blood that has built up or the stitches dissolving (this depends on the type of stitches used and how fast they dissolve), but sometimes it can be an indicator that you have overdone it somewhat.  You may also experience some sort of vaginal discharge for a number of weeks as well.  The key with both is to see your

GP if they continue for longer than six to eight weeks or if they change significantly or are accompanied by other symptoms.

## 71. Slow down, and appreciate the day

So how are you going to fix it so that you take things easy for the first couple of weeks? I've already talked about being trying to be superwoman before the operation, now what about being super-relaxed after? What do you think is going to really get on your nerves if it's not done? Making the bed, keeping the bathroom clean or weeding the garden?

Whatever it is sort out a way to get round it before you go into hospital by asking family and friends to help out. Stress and worry will ensure that you don't heal as quickly as you could; relaxation and enjoying the moment will.

How tired you feel after your hysterectomy is going to come as a shock and taking the time to do nothing is one of the best gifts you can give yourself. You will be up and about and feeling fitter, much sooner than if you try to push yourself too early. So, give yourself a break and make getting better the most important 'job' you can do right now.

## 72. Side effects of hysterectomy (i) ✑

There are many possible symptoms that you might experience after a hysterectomy; you may have many or none at all. I've listed the most commonly reported so that you can be aware of what is and isn't normal.

And do remember that most women say it takes up to six months before they are no longer thinking about having had a hysterectomy on a daily basis, and many will say it takes one to two years to fully recover.

⊛ Incredible tiredness, can last for two or three months, increasing your activity levels helps.

⊛ Frequency and urgency of urination could be due to infection or irritation by the catheter

⊛ Pain around any wound, this can be localized as well

⊛ Discharge or weeping around any wound in the first week or two

⊛ Itching or burning around any wound

⊛ Lack or sensation or numbness on one or both sides of the groin or legs

⊛ Swelling around any wound

⊛ Bloating and wind

⊛ Constipation or diarrhoea (if you had antibiotics)

⊛ Vaginal discharge and/or smell (both may require some sort of antibiotic)

⊛ Burning or itching around the vulva (this is usually due to dryness and not yeast infection)

⊛ Pain and swelling or redness at the site of the intravenous needles

⊛ Pelvic cramps which may be related to increased physical activity

## 73. Pet therapy

Research has shown that heart attack victims who have pets live longer. Even watching a tank full of tropical fish may lower blood pressure, at least temporarily. It is known that pet ownership affects people physiologically, and psychologically, as the soothing, relaxing effect of stroking or sitting with a pet slows your heart rate down. Pets are also wonderful to have around when you aren't feeling well as they often sense what you need and will be there for you; no need to talk, no need to explain, all you need to do, is 'be'.

Of course if you have a pet you're also going to have to think of some of the practicalities, especially if you live alone. Will you book Harry into the local kennels or can a friend have Tom for you (apologies to those of you with a partner called Harry or Tom!). Can you persuade a friend to pick up the pet food on the weekly shop and a dog walker can be a fantastic investment after you get home from hospital as you won't have to worry about walking further than you're able to, or being pulled over.

## 74. Looking after your wound ☺ ⓘ ✓

You may well have a large abdominal wound after your hysterectomy and it is going to be important to look after it well until it has completely healed. Your wound will begin healing immediately after your hysterectomy and it is important to promote this by keeping it (and any dressings) clean and dry until it has begun to heal properly.

You may experience some discharge from the site of your wound although this could well be a normal part of your healing process. If you do get an infection then you will probably be prescribed some antibiotics or an antiseptic cream to use as directed by your GP.

After your wound has healed, rubbing Calendula cream into the scar will help the skin to remain supple and prevent puckering. The skin on the scar is going to be fragile for quite a long time and most surgeons will also recommend that you avoid direct sunlight on the newly formed scar tissue. So there'll be no flashing it around on the beach in Marbella this year.

## 75. Write a poem to your womb ☺

There is every chance that your hysterectomy will be one of the most liberating experiences you will have. It could end years of symptoms that have been painful and difficult to live with, but we should still acknowledge that it may also cause some emotional upheaval as well.

Part of the recovery after your operation is going to be about coming to terms with something that has dominated much of your life up until this point and you should not ignore its significance. You will also go through a natural grieving process and will experience some degree of shock, anger and resentment before adjusting and reaching a level of hope for a better future. The extent to which you feel these emotions will depend on many factors and there is no 'average' unfortunately.

Writing a poem to your womb, or your body in general, can help you to begin to express all of the feelings you have held about it over the years, and once they are out in the open you will be free to move on. So go on, tell it how you feel, tell it how much you have resented the problems it has caused, thank it for any children you have given birth to and finally tell it about how much you are going to enjoy your bright future.

## 76. Aromatherapy

Aromatherapy is a truly holistic therapy that takes into account the whole person. It acts on many senses at once and can be used to induce both healing and relaxation.

You can use the oils in many different ways; put them into oil burners to benefit from the aroma, add small quantities to your bath water (but do remember to keep any wounds and dressings dry), massage them into your skin as long as they are diluted with carrier oil or you could use them in a compress. But under no circumstances should you drink them.

Those that you might find most beneficial after a hysterectomy include some with antibacterial properties such as Tea Tree, Lavender, Eucalyptus, Bergamot and Juniper. Jasmine, Bergamot, Geranium, Lavender and Ylang

Ylang can all lift your mood and if you would like to give your sex life a boost, then Ylang Ylang, Rose and Neroli are the ones to go for. Geranium also balances hormones and Clary Sage, Fennel, Star Anise and Tarragon have some oestrogenic qualities which may be useful for managing menopausal symptoms.

### 77. Healing laughter

It beats almost any pill or potion as laughing out loud releases a surge of 'feel good' hormones and a rush of energy that reduces fatigue and tension, slashes the production of stress hormones, boosts the immune system and protects the heart.

There is a health warning though, it can be painful in those early days after your hysterectomy, so put your recovery cushion over your tummy and wrap your arms around it to hold your muscles firmly.

So how do you rate yourself? Have you got the necessary GSOH (good sense of humour) required to respond to the dating advert in the local paper? When was the last time you had a good belly-laugh? What makes you laugh? Are you a naturally humorous person? Can you start laughing now?

Make a list of the top ten things that get you chuckling, be they books, videos, magazines or your private hoard of recollections. Don't leave this handy hint until you've made the list; once you've experienced the effects, you'll want to include laughter as an essential part of your daily recovery diet.

## 78. Phyto-oestrogen's 😊 🌓 ✍

So what are phyto-oestrogens?  Well they are chemicals of plant origin that mimic the action of the female hormone, oestrogen.  Recent research has suggested that they can be helpful in reducing the severity of some menopausal symptoms[18], such as hot flushes and night sweats.  By supplementing the diet of some volunteers with Soya beans, Red Clover and Linseed oil, researchers found that the women's levels of FSH (Follicle Stimulating Hormone) which increases after the menopause, actually reduced to pre-menopausal levels.  It is believed that this is why women in Japan, who have diets high in Soya, are less likely to have menopausal symptoms at all.

Other sources of phyto-oestrogens include whole grains, chickpeas, lentils, garlic, celery, rhubarb, alfalfa sprouts and parsley.

Perhaps the easiest way to take phyto-oestrogens is by increasing the amount of Soya you eat.  You could do this by adding Soya yoghurt and milk to your diet, or even by substituting some of your usual flour for Soya flour when, and if, you bake.  Your local health food store also probably stocks many supplements containing Red Clover, Linseed and Soya.

## 79. Rest and recuperation 😊 ✍ ✔

Resting is one of the hardest things for many women to do, but rest you must if you want to recover as quickly and easily as is possible.  There are many different types of rest but one of the most important is bed rest, in particular sleeping.

Research has shown that during Non REM (dreamless) sleep the body repairs and regenerates tissues, builds bone and muscle, and appears to strengthen the immune system, while REM (dreaming) sleep acts as a psychological safety valve, helping us work through unconscious events and emotional issues.

In addition to sleeping, being in bed and lying down means that you won't be putting a strain on the surgery site.    If you've had your cervix removed then the vaginal area will also need time to heal without having the pressure of the remaining abdominal organs bearing down on it.

So the key ladies, is to rest in bed as much as you can, for as long as you can and when you get bored, get up and get moving; then potter back to bed again for a few hours of helpful, restorative sleep.


## 80. The healing properties of honey

Honey has long been thought to have many positive healing qualities and in recent years it has been enjoying something of a revival in wound care for skin abscesses as it acts as an antibacterial and antifungal agent and helps to disinfect the skin and speed up the healing process.    It has a huge range of unique nutritional and health benefits, too many to be listed here, although researchers in California have now shown that eating honey can also raise the levels of anti-oxidants in the body.

Manuka Honey, specifically, is used to inhibit the growth of helicobacter pylori the bacteria that is implicated in many stomach ulcers.

As well as all of these benefits, honey is also a healthier option than white sugar, mainly because it is a more complex sugar, you don't need to use as much of it and it is at least one quarter water.    If you like the idea of honey, you could add it to herbal and fruit teas, or put a nice big dollop on top of some Greek yoghurt, for a traditional Greek dessert.

## 81. Showers vs baths ✍

A hysterectomy is definitely going to make you less flexible for a few weeks, you will find it difficult to bend, and getting up and down from a chair can become a marathon.  So rather than trying to make life difficult, use the shower instead of the bath, they are so much easier to get out of.  As well as this wonderful sense of ease, it will be easier to keep your wound and any dressings clean and dry.

But what happens if you don't have a shower?  Perhaps investing in a hand held shower spray might be a good idea, at least that way you can sit on the side of the bath to wash yourself with a face cloth.  If this still isn't an option and you have no choice but to use a bath then it might be worth spending a little time before your operation working out how you're going to get in and out and whether you have enough room around you to do it comfortably.  You must remember though, that the water should not come up to any wounds until they have healed well.

Once any wounds have healed and you have become more flexible, then the warm water of a bath can be a wonderful way to relax, but remember don't add any bath oils or bubbles until you are healed completely; you don't want to undo all the good you've already done.


## 82. Menopause Cake ☺ ✍

This is my own version of a cake that was originally developed by Linda Kearns who was tired of taking HRT and who wanted to try to reduce her menopausal symptoms more naturally.  Convinced that phyto-oestrogens were the way to go she formulated a recipe that would provide her with the optimal daily amount of Soya and Linseed.

- 100g (4oz) soy flour
- 100g (4oz) whole-wheat flour
- 1pc stem ginger finely chopped
- 100g (4oz) porridge oats
- 100g (4oz) raisins
- 1 ripe peeled banana
- 50g (2oz) sunflower seeds
- 50g (2oz) cup flaked almonds
- 50g (2ozg) sesame seeds
- 50g (2oz) pumpkin seeds
- 100g (4oz) linseeds
- ½ tsp ground ginger
- ½ tsp cinnamon
- ½ teaspoon nutmeg
- ¾ litre (900ml) soymilk

Put all the dry ingredients in a large mixing bowl. Add the Soya milk, mix well and leave to soak for about 30 minutes. Heat the oven to 190°C. Line a small loaf tin with waxed paper. If the mixture ends up too stiff or too thick to pour, stir in some more Soya milk. Spoon the mixture into the baking tin and bake for 1½ hours. Test with a skewer and if it is not cooked through, allow five to ten more minutes. Turn out on a wire rack to cool. It is delicious with butter or on its own; ideally you should eat one slice a day. If you don't want to make your own, you can also buy Linda Kearn's cake from *www.bake-it.com.* Just one slice contains the RDA of phyto-estrogens.

### 83. Bowel cleansing drink

If you are having problems with constipation, perhaps because you have some pain, or fear of pain, then this is the drink for you.

- 1 small bottle prune juice
- 1 small apple, peeled, cored and chopped
- 1 small teaspoon linseeds
- ½ litre sparkling mineral water

Put all of the ingredients in your blender and whiz on full power for a couple of minutes, pour into a jug and keep in the fridge for the day, drinking a small glass in the morning, afternoon and evening together with plenty of plain water, until it works!.

## 84. The value of big knickers ☺ ✍ ✔

There is no doubt about it, this is one time in your life that you are really going to appreciate Big Knickers in a way you haven't done since you read or watched 'Bridget Jones'.

Any wounds you may have as well as your tummy muscles are all going to be very tender for quite a while and you really won't appreciate being rubbed by knicker elastic. So Big Knickers are going to be *'so this season'* that you really need to invest in a dozen pairs before your hysterectomy takes place. Make sure that they come well up to your waist and they aren't a size too small, this is no time for vanity ladies. Under no circumstances think about going for a thong right now, they're going to be just far too painful. Treat your tummy kindly, it'll repay you in a few weeks time.

# My Notes

# In the long term

## 85. Take a holiday

This holiday is elevated to a prescriptive, therapeutic necessity for you. It's time for indulgence.

So what is your ideal holiday?  Do you want a whole week of relaxing on a beach and lying in the sun being waited on? Or would that drive you mad because you'd far rather be out exploring.  How about a combination of the two, according to how you felt that day?

It is possible that the health problems leading to your hysterectomy have impacted on your choice of holiday in the past to a greater or lesser extent. What will it be like to travel to exotic destinations and wear what you like around the pool?  Have new horizons opened up that were impossible in the past?

Holidays are also a great opportunity to revitalise your relationship, and what better place to do it than at the poolside with a glass of wine in one hand and who knows what in the other.

If you do plan a holiday that means you need to travel by air or sea, you may need to find out from your travel insurance company whether there are any restrictions within your policy.  They can also give you guidance about when they feel it is appropriate to travel.

## 86. Give a little back

If you've done all the things suggested in this book, then one hint you might have enjoyed particularly was spending time some on internet forums.

Now that you are almost recovered and have all that experience behind you, why not consider using it, for a time, to help other women who might be as concerned and nervous as you once were. Not only will it help you put your experience into perspective, but it will be a tremendous help for others.

If you did have a difficult time, talk about it and share what did, and didn't, work for you. You can almost guarantee that someone, somewhere, sometime, is going to thank you for donating those pearls of wisdom to the world. In the same way, if you've had a good experience, talk about it and shout it from the rooftops.

And last of all, what about sending us your own hints and tips and we will add them to our free emails.


## 87. Change of life or change your life?

Psychotherapists regard hysterectomy and the menopause as major life stages for a woman. When the menopause occurs at the same time as other significant life events, it often becomes a time for reflection on the past and a rethink on where you're going. Would you like life to stay very much as it is, or are there some things you'd like to change. Have you got things on a 'must do' list, that are undone? Have you got any dreams or passions that life and health had made impossible until now?

You've got to take it easy physically for the next few weeks, so in your hysterectomy journal answer the question "what is the meaning of life", then have a short rest before you get started!


## 88. Returning to work

The standard answer often given for a return to work is usually six to eight weeks, but of course this is dependent on so many different factors. Answering the following questions may help you make some decisions.

---

⊛ What type of operation did you have?

⊛ Why did you have a hysterectomy?

⊛ How ill were you before your operation?

⊛ How do you get to work, by bus, car or walking?

⊛ What type of work do you do?

⊛ How much support you have had at home during recovery?

---

For those in jobs that involve standing for long periods or where there is a lot of lifting, stretching or bending then a slightly longer period of recovery may be needed. Those who have desk jobs may be able to get back to work slightly sooner.

It is advisable to talk to your employer as soon as you are given a date for your operation as they may need to find temporary replacement and you will also need to check your entitlement to sick pay. If you are a manager then it could be useful to prepare your staff to cover for you, and if you are self employed, you will need to let your clients know that you won't be around for a while.

When you do go back to work, it might be possible to talk to your employer about doing reduced hours or a different job for a few weeks. For those that really can't keep away, what about seeing if you can do some work at home.

Keeping in touch with the personnel department and your line manager while you are away will keep you up to date with everything that is happening and you can keep them informed about how you're doing. Do remember though to be realistic about what you can, and can't, do.

## 89. Managing weight gain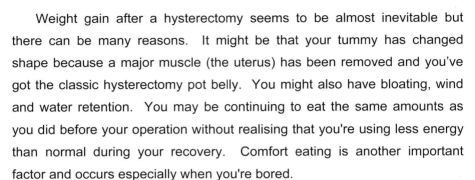

Weight gain after a hysterectomy seems to be almost inevitable but there can be many reasons. It might be that your tummy has changed shape because a major muscle (the uterus) has been removed and you've got the classic hysterectomy pot belly. You might also have bloating, wind and water retention. You may be continuing to eat the same amounts as you did before your operation without realising that you're using less energy than normal during your recovery. Comfort eating is another important factor and occurs especially when you're bored.

Ultimately the only way to lose weight is to use more energy than you are putting in, so a gentle increase in your daily activity levels should be very helpful.

But, having said all that, you have just had a major operation and you are entitled to indulge and pamper yourself for a while.

## 90. Learn belly dancing

I know that when you read this, the last thing you are going to want to try is belly dancing, but belly dancing (or Raks Sharqi as it is also called) works with the body, not against it. The graceful hip drops, rolls, and pivots use many of the muscle groups in the abdomen, pelvis, trunk, spine, and neck and of course such movements come naturally to the female form.

When you're feeling better and looking for some gentle exercise, it could be worth finding out if there is a local class as the movements will tone the muscles and help maintain your flexibility in a safe and effective way. It can also help prevent lower back problem, tone up your arms and shoulders and, as it is weight bearing, can help to prevent osteoporosis.

As well as all of these benefits, you can use up to 300 calories an hour at a class. So if you have some extra weight to shift then this could be the exercise for you. But, before you do anything, check with your GP that it's okay for you to start, you don't want to overdo it now do you?

## 91. Tai Chi, Yoga and Pilates ☺

There are many types of exercise which you can begin a couple of months after your hysterectomy that are gentle and which will gradually help to tone your body up. Some of the best are Tai Chi, Yoga and Pilates. Each of them focuses on moving the body slowly through a series of specific movements while concentrating on your breathing as you are doing them. They are perfect for beginners at exercise as well as those who are somewhat fitter.

In addition because they are specific movements, teachers concentrate on making sure you do them correctly so that you place as little strain as possible on joints and muscles which prevents injury.

All of them work on improving relaxation, stamina, coordination, breathing, concentration, strength, body alignment and general fitness. Before you start a class though, it is best to let the teacher know that you've recently had major surgery, so that they can take that into account when asking you to do the movements.

## 92. Getting behind the steering wheel ⓘ ✍ ✔

Some hospital information leaflets recommend that you wait six weeks after hysterectomy before you try driving again. Some may even vary the timescale according to the type of hysterectomy you had. However, (are you getting tired of me saying this yet?), you're the expert on your body and there are five things to consider, together with any other general recommendations made by the hospital. You may be surprised by how your much you use your abdominal muscles when driving.

---

⊛ You need to be able to use the clutch, accelerator and brake

⊛ You must be able to do an emergency stop without hesitation

⊛ Check the requirements of your insurance policy

⊛ You must be able to turn your head to see behind you for reversing

⊛ Keep the drive short for the first few times and take a friend with you.

---

## 93. About sex ☯ ✎ ✓

You're unique, did you know that? Although the hospital leaflet may have suggested you refrain from sex for six weeks, only you will know whether the time is right. At around the six-week mark, there should be no pain in your genitals or abdomen, the wound should have healed, and any discharge should have stopped. You may also feel emotionally ready.

For weeks, months or years before your hysterectomy, you may have associated sex with discomfort and pain. But now this is the new you. Set the scene with warmth, no interruptions guaranteed, maybe an ylang-ylang room fragrance, a little mood lighting and a bottle of essential oil for massage and finally, your most precious gift of time. Take plenty of it; let your partner make sure you are well lubricated, either naturally or with KY Jelly, and enjoy. If you're worried about the depth of penetration or anticipate pain, then girls on top might be a treat for both of you and it will allow you to ensure you're comfortable. And afterwards, cuddle up close and make plans for your new life ahead.

## 94. Spa's 4 U ❗

So you're finally about to go back to work. You're feeling pretty good considering but lets face it you could really do with just one more bit of 'me' time. If you can afford it, book yourself into a spa for the day and just indulge in a massage, a facial, good food and relaxation.

But I guess most of you won't want to do that and doing it at home can be just as much fun. If you have children, persuade someone to have them for you for the day and book yourself in for a haircut; remember you gave yourself that new look just before your operation? Why not get a manicure and pedicure done at the same time?

When you get home light some candles in the bathroom, run a warm bath and add some delicious bath oils to soften the skin, put some relaxing music on the stereo (just loud enough for you to hear in the bathroom). Finally turn the lights out, or down, and slip into the bath and lie quietly for an hour or so. When you get out, dry yourself off and rub in plenty of body lotion and then wrap yourself up in a bathrobe and settle down on the sofa with a glass of wine and your favourite book or video; bliss. Who knows, you may even make this a regular event.

## 95. Burn the tampons ☺

So what are the best bits about having had a hysterectomy? I would guess that one them has to be having no more sanitary towels or tampons to deal with. One woman wrote and said that on her trips to the supermarket after she had recovered, she would skip past the sanitary towel aisle, safe in the knowledge that she wouldn't have to go through anything like that again. And being creative with how you dispose of your remaining sanitary products and contraceptives is one way of demonstrating the very powerful change that has been wrought through your hysterectomy. Change for the better for the vast majority of women.

Since you hit puberty, your body has been ruled by hormones, your period pains and bleeding as well as all the other symptoms that led you to the point of having a hysterectomy. Well, its time to let go of all the negative stuff and really rejoice in the future. Just think you're no longer tied to your periods, no more limiting life styles that stop you from doing all the things that you want to do, like abseiling down the front of the office building or leaping out of a plane at 10,000 feet. The sky is now your limit and you can enjoy the life you were always meant to have.

What about hosting a barbeque and use your spare tampons and pads as briquettes, or you could build a bonfire. Either way, using fire to say 'out with the old' is extremely symbolic.

Alternatively you could do something fun, like making Suney's Tampon Angels – find out how at: *web.dbtech.net/~suncastl/angel.htm*. In fact why not get your girlfriends in and make a party of it with some wine and nibbles; at the very least you'll have a laugh. (P.S. I'd recommend dipping in water and hanging them up by the string the day before the party).

If none of these are for you, or if you have huge stocks, why not see if your local hospital or nursing home might like them instead.

Now, every time you go to your local supermarket, glide down the sanitary towel aisle and say "thank you for the extra days I have a month".

## 96. Biorhythms

As you know, the human body is governed by a number of a natural rhythms and biological cycles, like the menstrual cycle. Biorhythm theory suggests that internal cycles regulate our internal emotional, physical and intellectual functions. Everyone's biorhythms start at the moment of birth, with the physical aspect completing its cycle in twenty three days, the emotional in twenty eight days and the intellectual in thirty three days, before starting all over again. The only time all three cycles are at zero simultaneously again, is at the age of fifty eight years and sixty six days, an age which biorhythmists call 'rebirthing'.

Your biorhythms may help explain some of your mood changes and could also highlight days when your physical cycle is low and it might not be wise to try and run a marathon. So if you're feeling emotionally flat and low, quite negative with a lack of fresh ideas and feeling generally uncreative, check it out on any number of free websites and see if it works for you. You can find them by typing in the term 'biorhythms'.

## 97. Heart health ☺ ⓘ ✍ ✓

More women die of heart disease related illnesses than any other illness, and if you have a hysterectomy that removes your ovaries you will need to think about looking after your heart as this, together with your bones, is directly affected by the menopause and the consequent drop in oestrogen. You could take HRT, but if you don't want to do this, then the following dietary changes, supplements and complementary therapies might be beneficial to you.

---

⊛ Vitamin C, Vitamin E, essential fatty acids, beta-carotene

⊛ Ginkgo biloba, hawthorn, garlic and ginger

⊛ Regular aerobic exercise

⊛ Avoiding too much diary produce and red meat

⊛ Increasing your intake of fruit, vegetables, nuts, whole grains and seeds

---

## 98. Looking after your skin and hair

There is no doubt about it ageing affects the skin and hair noticeably. We all get wrinkles on our faces, more grey hairs appear every year and having major surgery will show up here as well. The menopause can precipitate skin and hair ageing and both your skin and hair may become drier and more fragile.

So what can you do about it? Well using a moisturiser and a good sunscreen to prevent prolonged exposure to the sun will help your skin; and conditioning treatments especially for dry hair will help it keep its lustre. You could also eat your way to good skin and hair, by eating plenty of eggs and liver for Vitamin A; dark green leafy vegetables, sweet potatoes and carrots for beta carotene; vegetable oils, nuts and seeds for your essential fatty acids and shellfish, red meat and pumpkin seeds for zinc. As well as all of these, drinking plenty of water is going to ensure that your skin looks full and plump and it will help your hair to be less dry and brittle.

Alternatively you could try one of the following natural remedies.

---

❀ Mix 2 tablespoons of honey with 2 teaspoons of whole milk, smooth over the face and throat, and let it moisturise your face for around 15 minutes. Rinse off with warm water and then splash with cold water.

❀ To give your hair a real shine, dissolve 1 teaspoon of honey into a large glass of warm water and use as a hair rinse. If you're blonde, add the juice of 1 lemon as well. Rinse well with warm water

---

## 99. Planning a recovery party

So how are you going to celebrate the new liberated you? You with the new life, new image and new positive outlook. What about a recovery party to say thanks to everyone that has helped you on the way to health; all those people who have done the dishes, got the shopping and been there to talk to and cry with.

Celebrate your success with a cake and sparkling wine. You could spend some of your recovery time thinking about the message you would like on the top of your cake, will it be funny or thought provoking?

So get your friends to bring the food, ask the supermarket to deliver the drinks, persuade everyone to bring their own glasses and plates (so you don't have to wash up after) and have fun, celebrating your health and happiness.

## 100. Getting a grip on your bones

After going through the menopause you may have an increased risk of osteoporosis as your hormone levels change over the next few years. One way of monitoring the strength of your bones is by regular (every three to four years) bone mineral densitometry tests that your GP can arrange for you. This scan will spot potentially harmful changes to your bone strength which means that appropriate action can then be taken.

You can also help yourself by taking moderate, regular bone strengthening exercise such as walking or running, and by changing to dietary habits that could contribute to your bone health.

⊛ Increase your levels of Vitamin D, calcium, magnesium and boron

⊛ Eat dark green leafy vegetables, fruit, whole grains and seeds

⊛ Add oily fish, baked beans and dried fruit to your diet

⊛ Avoid having too much red meat and coffee and stop smoking

# 101. Creative contraceptive disposal

You've done the pain, now let's have some fun! If you hadn't already gone through the menopause before your hysterectomy, the chances are you were probably still using some form of contraception and now you can finally dump them. What a relief, no more slippery caps flying all over the place, no more pills to take and no more condoms (unless safe sex is an issue).

Be creative with how you'll do the deed. If it's summer, and warm, what about water bombs in the garden? Finger puppets to amuse your most significant other are easy to make and with a few acrylic paints and crayons you can really let your alter-ego go. And how about a few balloons at your Recovery Party, of course you will need to be sure that your friends will share the joke and not be offended. You could practice Frisbee in the garden or use your cap as an interesting 'hat' the next time you need a fancy dress costume. If you've been taking the pill then the safest way to dispose of them is at your local chemists, you could even make it fun by putting them in brightly coloured gift bags with tags and perhaps a free lollipop before handing them over the counter!

Why not add your suggestions to the forums on The Hysterectomy Association website under "creative disposals".

*For even more handy hints and tips for a happy hysterectomy visit:*
*www.hysterectomy-association.org.uk*

# Appendices

# My Notes

# Scaling Diary

Day: ........................../ Date: ................................ / Time: ..........................

*(1 is the worst you've had or done and 10 is the best you've had or done)*

| ⊛ Pain | 1 | 2 | 3 | 4 | 5 | 6 | 7 | 8 | 9 | 10 |
|---|---|---|---|---|---|---|---|---|---|---|
| ⊛ Sleeping | 1 | 2 | 3 | 4 | 5 | 6 | 7 | 8 | 9 | 10 |
| ⊛ Mood | 1 | 2 | 3 | 4 | 5 | 6 | 7 | 8 | 9 | 10 |
| ⊛ Tiredness | 1 | 2 | 3 | 4 | 5 | 6 | 7 | 8 | 9 | 10 |
| ⊛ Walking/exercise | 1 | 2 | 3 | 4 | 5 | 6 | 7 | 8 | 9 | 10 |

Comments:

Day: ........................../ Date: ................................ / Time: ..........................

*(1 is the worst you've had or done and 10 is the best you've had or done)*

| ⊛ Pain | 1 | 2 | 3 | 4 | 5 | 6 | 7 | 8 | 9 | 10 |
|---|---|---|---|---|---|---|---|---|---|---|
| ⊛ Sleeping | 1 | 2 | 3 | 4 | 5 | 6 | 7 | 8 | 9 | 10 |
| ⊛ Mood | 1 | 2 | 3 | 4 | 5 | 6 | 7 | 8 | 9 | 10 |
| ⊛ Tiredness | 1 | 2 | 3 | 4 | 5 | 6 | 7 | 8 | 9 | 10 |
| ⊛ Walking/exercise | 1 | 2 | 3 | 4 | 5 | 6 | 7 | 8 | 9 | 10 |

Comments:

Day: ........................../ Date: ................................ / Time: ..........................

*(1 is the worst you've had or done and 10 is the best you've had or done)*

| ⊛ Pain | 1 | 2 | 3 | 4 | 5 | 6 | 7 | 8 | 9 | 10 |
|---|---|---|---|---|---|---|---|---|---|---|
| ⊛ Sleeping | 1 | 2 | 3 | 4 | 5 | 6 | 7 | 8 | 9 | 10 |
| ⊛ Mood | 1 | 2 | 3 | 4 | 5 | 6 | 7 | 8 | 9 | 10 |
| ⊛ Tiredness | 1 | 2 | 3 | 4 | 5 | 6 | 7 | 8 | 9 | 10 |
| ⊛ Walking/exercise | 1 | 2 | 3 | 4 | 5 | 6 | 7 | 8 | 9 | 10 |

Comments:

Day: ........................../ Date: ................................. / Time: ..........................

*(1 is the worst you've had or done and 10 is the best you've had or done)*

| ⊛ Pain | 1 | 2 | 3 | 4 | 5 | 6 | 7 | 8 | 9 | 10 |
|---|---|---|---|---|---|---|---|---|---|---|
| ⊛ Sleeping | 1 | 2 | 3 | 4 | 5 | 6 | 7 | 8 | 9 | 10 |
| ⊛ Mood | 1 | 2 | 3 | 4 | 5 | 6 | 7 | 8 | 9 | 10 |
| ⊛ Tiredness | 1 | 2 | 3 | 4 | 5 | 6 | 7 | 8 | 9 | 10 |
| ⊛ Walking/exercise | 1 | 2 | 3 | 4 | 5 | 6 | 7 | 8 | 9 | 10 |
| Comments: | | | | | | | | | | |

Day: ........................../ Date: ................................. / Time: ..........................

*(1 is the worst you've had or done and 10 is the best you've had or done)*

| ⊛ Pain | 1 | 2 | 3 | 4 | 5 | 6 | 7 | 8 | 9 | 10 |
|---|---|---|---|---|---|---|---|---|---|---|
| ⊛ Sleeping | 1 | 2 | 3 | 4 | 5 | 6 | 7 | 8 | 9 | 10 |
| ⊛ Mood | 1 | 2 | 3 | 4 | 5 | 6 | 7 | 8 | 9 | 10 |
| ⊛ Tiredness | 1 | 2 | 3 | 4 | 5 | 6 | 7 | 8 | 9 | 10 |
| ⊛ Walking/exercise | 1 | 2 | 3 | 4 | 5 | 6 | 7 | 8 | 9 | 10 |
| Comments: | | | | | | | | | | |

***Why not download an A4 sheet of these diaries from www.hysterectomy-association.org.uk/101resources.php***

# Step by Step to Recovery

| | |
|---|---|
| **Week 1**<br>after getting home from hospital | No household tasks at all<br>Lie on (or in) the bed as much as necessary<br>Sleep when you need to<br>Do as many of the light exercises as possible<br>Shower daily<br>Walk around the house 2-3 times daily – on one floor if possible<br>Lie down, rather than sit<br>Sit, rather than stand |
| **Week 2** | Lie on (or in) the bed as much as necessary<br>Rest for at least two hours per day<br>Avoid long periods of sitting or standing<br>Help with washing up/drying dishes – sitting down if possible<br>Sit down to prepare vegetables<br>Daily walk outside – 10 minutes per day<br>Walking around the house – 2-3 times daily, including stairs once<br>Boil just enough water for a mug in a kettle |
| **Week 3** | Increase your walking by a 2 minutes daily<br>Try using the stairs at home 2-3 times a day<br>Light shopping in immediate vicinity – ie magazine or newspaper<br>Boil enough water for 2 mugs in the kettle<br>If you have any pain – stop immediately |
| **Week 4** | Start walking further outdoors – up to 20 minutes twice a day<br>You can probably go out in the car by now |

| | |
|---|---|
| | Should be able to make tea and coffee for three people<br>Help with dusting |
| **Week 5-6** | Can probably start some light routine housework<br>May be able to drive a car<br>Can possibly use an upright vacuum cleaner<br>Try gentle pelvic floor exercises – stop if you feel pain<br>Try vacuuming with a cylinder cleaner (week 6-7)<br>Try bed making (but not changing duvets)<br>(with either, stop if you have pain) |

# Exercises for Recovery

There are a variety of exercises you can try for different stages of your recovery, I have grouped them here to make it easier to see what you should be doing and when.

| | |
|---|---|
| **Exercises To Do While You're In Hospital** | These exercises are designed to get your circulation moving and your muscles mobile again. They can all be done in bed, but remember if you feel too much pain – then you should stop. They are similar to exercises you might do when flying to help guard against DVT.<br><br>1.  rolling the ankles round in a circle<br>2.  curling your feet towards you<br>3.  stretching your feet away from you<br>4.  Breath in deeply for a count of five and breath out slowly for a count of five<br><br>Increase the number of times you do each of these as you feel stronger. |
| **Week 1 – 4**<br><br>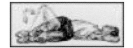 | Carry on with the hospital exercises whenever you are lying on the bed.<br><br>Lie on your back with your knees bent up, as if you were going to get out of bed. Allow the knees to drop first to one side, and then to the other.<br><br>Lie on your back with your knees bent up and press the middle of your back down into the mattress by pulling in your tummy muscles as hard as you can at this stage, tighten your buttocks at the same time. Hold as long as you can and then release.<br><br>Lie on your back with your knees resting on a pillow |

| | |
|---|---|
| | and your arms by your sides. Now gently stretch one arm towards your feet along the side of your body and then come back; repeat on the other side,<br><br>Gradually increase the number of times you do each of these exercises as your muscles get stronger. |
| **Weeks 5 - 7**<br>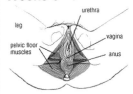 | Carry on with all the exercises listed in the previous weeks, increasing the number of repetitions you are doing daily.<br><br>Introduce the Kegel (Pelvic Floor Exercises). To locate the right muscles, next time you are on the loo, tighten your abdominal muscles so that the flow or urine stops. Count up to five and then release the flow. The aim is to prevent any leakage at all. You can repeat these exercises as much as your muscles are able to as they will help prevent possible future incontinence or prolapse.<br><br>Improve your abdominal muscles by lying on your back with your knees bent and then gently lift your head and shoulders off the floor (or bed) and reach your hands down towards your knees. |

# References

1.  Originally published on '*Songs by Tom Lehrer*', 1953

2.  *The International Aloe Science*, Council
http://www.iasc.org/articles.html

3.  Parker, W.H. & Parker, L. *A Gynaecologists Second Opinion*, 1996; p275

4.  Celso-Ramon Garcia, M.D. Winnifred B. Cutler, Ph.D. *Preservation of the Ovary: A Reevaluation*, Fertility and Sterility (Vol.42. No.4 October, 1984)

5.  Parker, W.H. & Parker, L. *A Gynaecologists Second Opinion*, 1996; p277

6.  Goldfarb, H.A. & Greif, J. *The No Hysterectomy Option*, 1997, pp147-148

7.  Parkinson-Hardman, L. *The Pocket Guide to Hysterectomy*, 2005, pp 52-53

8.  Davis, S.R. *The use of testosterone after menopause*, J Br Menopause Soc 2004 Jun;10(2): pp65-9

9.  Prasad A.S. et al, *Zinc status and serum testosterone levels of healthy adults*, Nutrition. 1996 May;12(5):344-8

10. Ernst E. *The benefits of Arnica: 16 case reports*, Homeopathy 2003 Oct;92(4): pp217-9

11. Lydeking-Olsen E. et al, *Soymilk or progesterone for prevention of bone loss--a 2 year randomized, placebo-controlled trial*, Eur J Nutr 2004 Aug;43(4): pp246-57

12. Seeger H. et al, *The effect of progesterone and synthetic progestins on serum- and estradiol-stimulated proliferation of human breast cancer cells*, Horm Metab Res 2003 Feb;35(2): pp76-80

13. Sandoval M. et al, *Anti-inflammatory and antioxidant activities of cat's claw (Uncaria tomentosa and Uncaria guianensis) are independent of their alkaloid content*, Phytomedicine 2002 May;9(4): pp325-37

14. Philp HA. *Hot flashes--a review of the literature on alternative and complementary treatment approaches*, Altern Med Rev 2003 Aug;8(3): pp284-302

15. Viereck V. et al, *Black cohosh: just another phytoestrogen?*, Trends Endocrinol Metab 2005 May 28

16. Chopin Lucks B. *Vitex agnus castus essential oil and menopausal balance: a research update*, Complement Ther Nurs Midwifery 2003 Aug;9(3): pp157-60

17. Tsuchiya J. et al, *Single-blind follow-up study on the effectiveness of a symbiotic preparation in irritable bowel syndrome*, Chin J Dig Dis 2004;5(4): pp169-7

18. Kronenberg F & Fugh-Berman A. *Complementary and alternative medicine for menopausal symptoms: a review of randomized, controlled trials*, Ann Intern Med 2002 Nov 19;137(10): pp805-13.

# Bibliography

Charlish, A. *Cleansing for Body and Spirit*, 2000, Haldane Mason Ltd

Clark, J. *Hysterectomy and the Alternatives*, Vermillion, 2000

Costantino, M. *The Detox Handbook*, 2003, S Webb and Son

Davis, P. *Aromatherapy An A-Z*, 1996, CW Daniel Company Limited

DeAngelo, D. *Sudden Menopause*, 2001, Newleaf

Gray, D. *Fresh Smoothies*, 2000, Chancellor Press

Glenville, M, *Natural Alternatives to HRT*, Kyle Cathie, 1997

Glenville, M. and Esson L. *Natural Alternatives to HRT Cookbook*, 2000, Kyle Cathie

Glenville, M. and Esson, L. *Healthy Eating for the Menopause*, 2004, Kyle Cathie

Glouberman, Dr D., *Life Choices, Life Changes*, 2003, Hodder and Stoughton

Goldfarb H.A. and Greif, J. *The No-Hysterectomy Option*, 1997, Wiley

Hay, L. *You Can Heal Your Life*, Hay House, 1984

Lerner, H.G. *The Dance of Intimacy*, 1989, Harper Collins

McWhirter, A. and Clasen, L. (ed) *Foods that Harm, foods that heal*, 2002, Readers Digest

Merson, S. Lift Off, *100 Tips to Energize*, 2003, MQ Publications

Miller, J. *Guide to Reflexology*, 2000, Caxton Editions

Parker, W. and Parker, R,L. *A Gynaecologists Second Opinion*, Plume/Penguin 1996

Parkinson-Hardman, L. *The Pocket Guide to Hysterectomy*, 2005, The Hysterectomy Association

Richardson, R. *Natural Superwoman*, 2003, Kyle Cathie

Robinson, Dr A. The Which Guide to Womens Health, 1996, Which Consumer Guides

Sexual Health (ed), 2002, Geddes and Grossett

Shealy C.N. (ed) The Compete Illustrated Encycolpeida of Alternative Healing Therapies, Element, 1999

Shepperson Mills, D. and Vernon, M. Endometriosis, A key to healing through nutrition, 1999, Element Books Limited

Simester, L. The Natural Health Bible, 2001, Quadrille Publishing

Tosh, C. Guide to Meditation, 2001, Caxton Editions

Webb, A. Hysterectomy a new horizon (leaflet)

Womens Health, (ed) 2000, Geddes and Grosset

# My Notes

# My Notes

# Do you need more?

I would like to invite you to continue your search for relevant information by joining on our website:

## *www.hysterectomy-association.org.uk*

- Share your worries, concerns and triumphs with other women
- Read the blog to find out more about the latest research
- Get the latest information about the alternatives that may be appropriate
- Join us and ask questions of experts, find a listening ear or call our helpline
- Join us our thriving Facebook community @
  *www.hysterectomy-association.org.uk/facebook.htm*
- Follow me on Twitter @
  *www.twitter.com/hysterlady*

For information about having Linda come and speak to your organisation or group, please contact: The Hysterectomy Association on 01305 755607 or by email on info@hysterectomy-association.org.uk

# My Notes